This planner belongs to

_____

If found, please contact

_____

_____

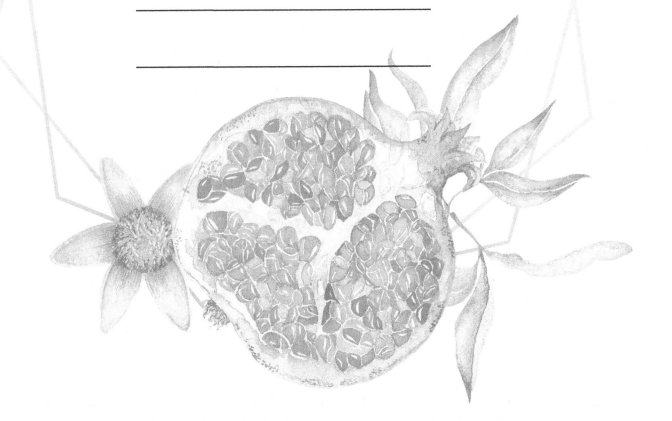

# What is a Flexitarian Diet?

As the name implies this is a 'flexible' diet that encourages you to eat more plant-based foods without becoming a total vegetarian.

It's the perfect combination for healthier eating, but still allows you to consume meat and diary products as you wish. This makes going out for dinner or attending a family function a little easier. On these days you can truly be 'flexible' with what you eat.

The guidelines for eating a Flexitarian Diet are:

- Eating mainly fruits, vegetables, legumes and whole grains
- Eat protein that is derived from plant protein
- Incorporate some meat and other animal products occasionally
- Eat mainly natural forms and avoid processed foods
- Be careful about adding sugars and eating too many sweets

That truly is all there is to it! Health benefits can include losing weight, reducing risk of heart disease and diabetes and possibly warding off certain cancers.

Please note that we are not qualified health professionals and always do your due diligence when it comes to changing your eating habits. Consult the advice of your doctor as needed.

# Suggested Foods

**Proteins:** Soybeans, tofu, tempeh, lentils, legumes
**Non-starchy vegetables:** All greens, bell peppers, Brussels sprouts, green beans, carrots, cauliflower, asparagus
**Starchy vegetables:** Winter squashes, peas, corn, sweet potato
**Fruits:** Apples, oranges, berries, grapes, cherries, bananas
**Whole grains:** Quinoa, buckwheat, brown rice
**Nuts, seeds and other healthy fats:** Almonds, flaxseeds, chia seeds, walnuts, cashews, pistachios, peanut butter, avocados, olives, coconut
**Plant-based milk:** Almond milk, coconut, hemp and soymilk
**Herbs, spices and seasonings:** Basil, oregano, mint, thyme, cumin, turmeric, ginger
**Condiments:** Reduced-sodium soy sauce, apple cider vinegar, salsa, mustard, nutritional yeast, ketchup sugar free
**Beverages:** Water, herbal tea, coffee organic

When using animal products, select from the following when possible:
**Eggs:** Free-range or grass fed
**Poultry:** Organic, free-range or grass fed
**Fish:** Wild-caught
**Meat:** Grass fed
**Dairy:** Organic from grass-fed

# Weekly Meal Planner

Week

|  | Breakfast | Lunch | Dinner | Snacks | Other |
|---|---|---|---|---|---|
| Monday | | | | | |
| Tuesday | | | | | |
| Wednesday | | | | | |
| Thursday | | | | | |
| Friday | | | | | |
| Saturday | | | | | |
| Sunday | | | | | |

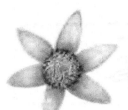

# Weekly Meal Planner

Week

|  | Breakfast | Lunch | Dinner | Snacks | Other |
|---|---|---|---|---|---|
| Monday | | | | | |
| Tuesday | | | | | |
| Wednesday | | | | | |
| Thursday | | | | | |
| Friday | | | | | |
| Saturday | | | | | |
| Sunday | | | | | |

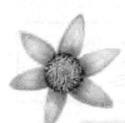

# Weekly Meal Planner

Week

|  | Breakfast | Lunch | Dinner | Snacks | Other |
|---|---|---|---|---|---|
| Monday |  |  |  |  |  |
| Tuesday |  |  |  |  |  |
| Wednesday |  |  |  |  |  |
| Thursday |  |  |  |  |  |
| Friday |  |  |  |  |  |
| Saturday |  |  |  |  |  |
| Sunday |  |  |  |  |  |

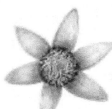

# Weekly Meal Planner

Week

|  | Breakfast | Lunch | Dinner | Snacks | Other |
|---|---|---|---|---|---|
| Monday | | | | | |
| Tuesday | | | | | |
| Wednesday | | | | | |
| Thursday | | | | | |
| Friday | | | | | |
| Saturday | | | | | |
| Sunday | | | | | |

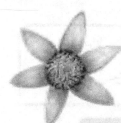

# Weekly Meal Planner

Week

|  | Breakfast | Lunch | Dinner | Snacks | Other |
|---|---|---|---|---|---|
| Monday | | | | | |
| Tuesday | | | | | |
| Wednesday | | | | | |
| Thursday | | | | | |
| Friday | | | | | |
| Saturday | | | | | |
| Sunday | | | | | |

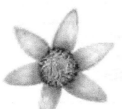

# Weekly Meal Planner

Week

|  | Breakfast | Lunch | Dinner | Snacks | Other |
|---|---|---|---|---|---|
| Monday |  |  |  |  |  |
| Tuesday |  |  |  |  |  |
| Wednesday |  |  |  |  |  |
| Thursday |  |  |  |  |  |
| Friday |  |  |  |  |  |
| Saturday |  |  |  |  |  |
| Sunday |  |  |  |  |  |

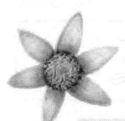

# Weekly Meal Planner

Week

|  | Breakfast | Lunch | Dinner | Snacks | Other |
|---|---|---|---|---|---|
| Monday | | | | | |
| Tuesday | | | | | |
| Wednesday | | | | | |
| Thursday | | | | | |
| Friday | | | | | |
| Saturday | | | | | |
| Sunday | | | | | |

# Weekly Meal Planner

Week

|  | Breakfast | Lunch | Dinner | Snacks | Other |
|---|---|---|---|---|---|
| Monday |  |  |  |  |  |
| Tuesday |  |  |  |  |  |
| Wednesday |  |  |  |  |  |
| Thursday |  |  |  |  |  |
| Friday |  |  |  |  |  |
| Saturday |  |  |  |  |  |
| Sunday |  |  |  |  |  |

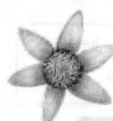

# Weekly Meal Planner

Week

|  | Breakfast | Lunch | Dinner | Snacks | Other |
|---|---|---|---|---|---|
| Monday | | | | | |
| Tuesday | | | | | |
| Wednesday | | | | | |
| Thursday | | | | | |
| Friday | | | | | |
| Saturday | | | | | |
| Sunday | | | | | |

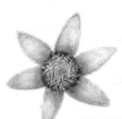

# Weekly Meal Planner

Week

|  | Breakfast | Lunch | Dinner | Snacks | Other |
|---|---|---|---|---|---|
| Monday |  |  |  |  |  |
| Tuesday |  |  |  |  |  |
| Wednesday |  |  |  |  |  |
| Thursday |  |  |  |  |  |
| Friday |  |  |  |  |  |
| Saturday |  |  |  |  |  |
| Sunday |  |  |  |  |  |

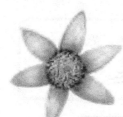

# Weekly Meal Planner

**Week**

|  | Breakfast | Lunch | Dinner | Snacks | Other |
|---|---|---|---|---|---|
| Monday |  |  |  |  |  |
| Tuesday |  |  |  |  |  |
| Wednesday |  |  |  |  |  |
| Thursday |  |  |  |  |  |
| Friday |  |  |  |  |  |
| Saturday |  |  |  |  |  |
| Sunday |  |  |  |  |  |

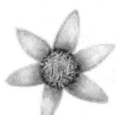

# Weekly Meal Planner

Week

|  | Breakfast | Lunch | Dinner | Snacks | Other |
|---|---|---|---|---|---|
| Monday | | | | | |
| Tuesday | | | | | |
| Wednesday | | | | | |
| Thursday | | | | | |
| Friday | | | | | |
| Saturday | | | | | |
| Sunday | | | | | |

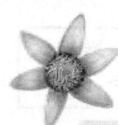

# Weekly Meal Planner

Week

|  | Breakfast | Lunch | Dinner | Snacks | Other |
|---|---|---|---|---|---|
| Monday | | | | | |
| Tuesday | | | | | |
| Wednesday | | | | | |
| Thursday | | | | | |
| Friday | | | | | |
| Saturday | | | | | |
| Sunday | | | | | |

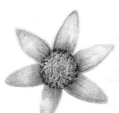

# Weekly Meal Planner

Week

|  | Breakfast | Lunch | Dinner | Snacks | Other |
|---|---|---|---|---|---|
| Monday | | | | | |
| Tuesday | | | | | |
| Wednesday | | | | | |
| Thursday | | | | | |
| Friday | | | | | |
| Saturday | | | | | |
| Sunday | | | | | |

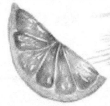

# Weekly Grocery List

Week

- ○
- ○
- ○
- ○
- ○
- ○

- ○
- ○
- ○
- ○
- ○
- ○

- ○
- ○
- ○
- ○
- ○
- ○

- ○
- ○
- ○
- ○
- ○
- ○

- ○
- ○
- ○
- ○
- ○
- ○

- ○
- ○
- ○
- ○
- ○
- ○

- ○
- ○
- ○
- ○
- ○

- ○
- ○
- ○
- ○
- ○

- ○
- ○
- ○
- ○
- ○

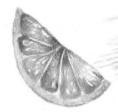

# Weekly Grocery List

Week

- ○ 
- ○ 
- ○ 
- ○ 
- ○ 
- ○ 
- ○ 
- ○ 
- ○ 
- ○ 
- ○ 
- ○ 
- ○ 
- ○ 
- ○ 
- ○ 
- ○ 
- ○ 
- ○ 
- ○ 
- ○

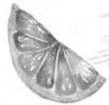

# Weekly Grocery List

Week

- ○ _____
- ○ _____
- ○ _____
- ○ _____
- ○ _____
- ○ _____

- ○ _____
- ○ _____
- ○ _____
- ○ _____
- ○ _____
- ○ _____

- ○ _____
- ○ _____
- ○ _____
- ○ _____
- ○ _____
- ○ _____

- ○ _____
- ○ _____
- ○ _____
- ○ _____
- ○ _____
- ○ _____

- ○ _____
- ○ _____
- ○ _____
- ○ _____
- ○ _____
- ○ _____

- ○ _____
- ○ _____
- ○ _____
- ○ _____
- ○ _____
- ○ _____

- ○ _____
- ○ _____
- ○ _____
- ○ _____
- ○ _____

- ○ _____
- ○ _____
- ○ _____
- ○ _____
- ○ _____

- ○ _____
- ○ _____
- ○ _____
- ○ _____
- ○ _____

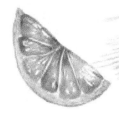

# Weekly Grocery List

Week

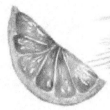

# Weekly Grocery List

Week

- ○
- ○
- ○
- ○
- ○
- ○

- ○
- ○
- ○
- ○
- ○

- ○
- ○
- ○
- ○
- ○

- ○
- ○
- ○
- ○
- ○
- ○

- ○
- ○
- ○
- ○
- ○
- ○

- ○
- ○
- ○
- ○
- ○
- ○

- ○
- ○
- ○
- ○
- ○

- ○
- ○
- ○
- ○
- ○

- ○
- ○
- ○
- ○
- ○

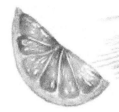

# Weekly Grocery List

Week

- ○
- ○
- ○
- ○
- ○
- ○
- ○
- ○
- ○
- ○
- ○
- ○
- ○
- ○
- ○
- ○
- ○
- ○
- ○
- ○
- ○

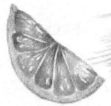

# Weekly Grocery List

Week

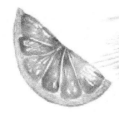

# Weekly Grocery List

Week

- ○
- ○
- ○
- ○
- ○
- ○
- ○
- ○
- ○
- ○
- ○
- ○
- ○
- ○
- ○
- ○
- ○
- ○
- ○
- ○

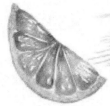

# Weekly Grocery List

**Week**

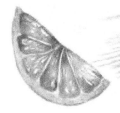

# Weekly Grocery List

Week

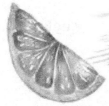

# Weekly Grocery List

Week

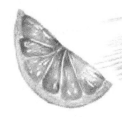 # Weekly Grocery List

**Week**

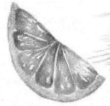

# Weekly Grocery List

**Week**

- ○
- ○
- ○
- ○
- ○
- ○

- ○
- ○
- ○
- ○
- ○
- ○

- ○
- ○
- ○
- ○
- ○
- ○

- ○
- ○
- ○
- ○
- ○
- ○

- ○
- ○
- ○
- ○
- ○
- ○

- ○
- ○
- ○
- ○
- ○
- ○

- ○
- ○
- ○
- ○
- ○

- ○
- ○
- ○
- ○
- ○

- ○
- ○
- ○
- ○
- ○

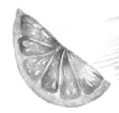

# Weekly Grocery List

Week

- ○
- ○
- ○
- ○
- ○
- ○
- ○
- ○
- ○
- ○
- ○
- ○
- ○
- ○
- ○
- ○
- ○
- ○
- ○
- ○
- ○
- ○

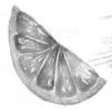

# Weekly Grocery List

**Week**

- ○
- ○
- ○
- ○
- ○
- ○

- ○
- ○
- ○
- ○
- ○
- ○

- ○
- ○
- ○
- ○
- ○
- ○

- ○
- ○
- ○
- ○
- ○
- ○

- ○
- ○
- ○
- ○
- ○
- ○

- ○
- ○
- ○
- ○
- ○
- ○

- ○
- ○
- ○
- ○
- ○

- ○
- ○
- ○
- ○
- ○

- ○
- ○
- ○
- ○
- ○

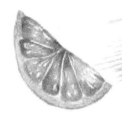

# Weekly Grocery List

Week

- ○
- ○
- ○
- ○
- ○
- ○
- ○
- ○
- ○
- ○
- ○
- ○
- ○
- ○
- ○
- ○
- ○
- ○
- ○
- ○
- ○

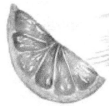

# Weekly Grocery List

**Week**

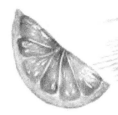

# Weekly Grocery List

Week

- ○
- ○
- ○
- ○
- ○
- ○
- ○
- ○
- ○
- ○
- ○
- ○
- ○
- ○
- ○
- ○
- ○
- ○
- ○
- ○

- ○
- ○
- ○
- ○
- ○
- ○
- ○
- ○
- ○
- ○
- ○
- ○
- ○
- ○
- ○
- ○
- ○
- ○
- ○
- ○

- ○
- ○
- ○
- ○
- ○
- ○
- ○
- ○
- ○
- ○
- ○
- ○
- ○
- ○
- ○
- ○
- ○
- ○
- ○
- ○

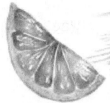

# Weekly Grocery List

Week

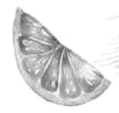

# Weekly Grocery List

Week

# Weekly Grocery List

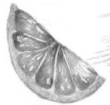

**Week**

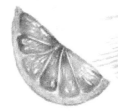

# Weekly Grocery List

Week

- ○
- ○
- ○
- ○
- ○
- ○
- ○
- ○
- ○
- ○
- ○
- ○
- ○
- ○
- ○
- ○
- ○
- ○
- ○

- ○
- ○
- ○
- ○
- ○
- ○
- ○
- ○
- ○
- ○
- ○
- ○
- ○
- ○
- ○
- ○
- ○
- ○
- ○

- ○
- ○
- ○
- ○
- ○
- ○
- ○
- ○
- ○
- ○
- ○
- ○
- ○
- ○
- ○
- ○
- ○
- ○
- ○

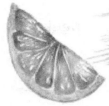

# Weekly Grocery List

**Week**

|  |  |  |
|---|---|---|
| ○ | ○ | ○ |
| ○ | ○ | ○ |
| ○ | ○ | ○ |
| ○ | ○ | ○ |
| ○ | ○ | ○ |
| ○ | ○ | ○ |

|  |  |  |
|---|---|---|
| ○ | ○ | ○ |
| ○ | ○ | ○ |
| ○ | ○ | ○ |
| ○ | ○ | ○ |
| ○ | ○ | ○ |
| ○ | ○ | ○ |

|  |  |  |
|---|---|---|
| ○ | ○ | ○ |
| ○ | ○ | ○ |
| ○ | ○ | ○ |
| ○ | ○ | ○ |
| ○ | ○ | ○ |

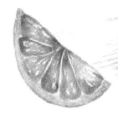

# Weekly Grocery List

Week

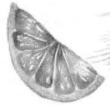

# Weekly Grocery List

Week

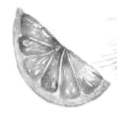

# Weekly Grocery List

Week

- ○ _____
- ○ _____
- ○ _____
- ○ _____
- ○ _____
- ○ _____
- ○ _____
- ○ _____
- ○ _____
- ○ _____
- ○ _____
- ○ _____
- ○ _____
- ○ _____
- ○ _____
- ○ _____
- ○ _____
- ○ _____
- ○ _____
- ○ _____

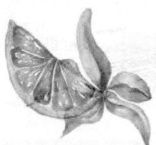

# Weekly Budget

Week

| Item | Budget | Actual |
|---|---|---|
| | | |

TOTAL

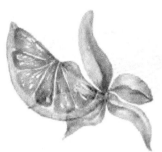

# Weekly Budget

Week

| Item | Budget | Actual |
|---|---|---|
| | | |
| | | |
| | | |
| | | |
| | | |
| | | |
| | | |
| | | |
| | | |
| | | |
| | | |
| | | |
| | | |
| | | |
| | | |
| | | |
| | | |
| | | |
| | | |
| | | |
| | | |
| | | |
| TOTAL | | |

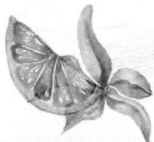

# Weekly Budget

**Week**

| Item | Budget | Actual |
|---|---|---|
|  |  |  |
|  |  |  |
|  |  |  |
|  |  |  |
|  |  |  |
|  |  |  |
|  |  |  |
|  |  |  |
|  |  |  |
|  |  |  |
|  |  |  |
|  |  |  |
|  |  |  |
|  |  |  |
|  |  |  |
|  |  |  |
|  |  |  |
|  |  |  |
|  |  |  |
|  |  |  |
|  |  |  |
|  | **TOTAL** |  |

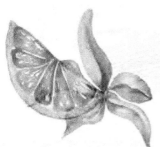

# Weekly Budget

Week

| Item | Budget | Actual |
|---|---|---|
| | | |
| | | |
| | | |
| | | |
| | | |
| | | |
| | | |
| | | |
| | | |
| | | |
| | | |
| | | |
| | | |
| | | |
| | | |
| | | |
| | | |
| | | |
| | | |
| | | |
| | | |
| | | |
| | | |
| | | |
| **TOTAL** | | |

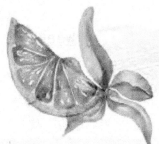

# Weekly Budget

Week

| Item | Budget | Actual |
|---|---|---|
| | | |
| | | |
| | | |
| | | |
| | | |
| | | |
| | | |
| | | |
| | | |
| | | |
| | | |
| | | |
| | | |
| | | |
| | | |
| | | |
| | | |
| | | |
| | | |
| | | |
| | | |
| **TOTAL** | | |

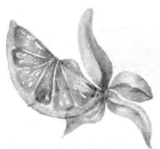

# Weekly Budget

Week

| Item | Budget | Actual |
|---|---|---|
| | | |
| | | |
| | | |
| | | |
| | | |
| | | |
| | | |
| | | |
| | | |
| | | |
| | | |
| | | |
| | | |
| | | |
| | | |
| | | |
| | | |
| | | |
| | | |
| | | |
| | | |
| | | |
| | | |
| | | |
| **TOTAL** | | |

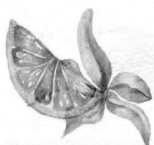

# Weekly Budget

Week

| Item | Budget | Actual |
|------|--------|--------|
|      |        |        |
|      |        |        |
|      |        |        |
|      |        |        |
|      |        |        |
|      |        |        |
|      |        |        |
|      |        |        |
|      |        |        |
|      |        |        |
|      |        |        |
|      |        |        |
|      |        |        |
|      |        |        |
|      |        |        |
|      |        |        |
|      |        |        |
|      |        |        |
|      |        |        |
|      |        |        |
|      |        |        |
| TOTAL |      |        |

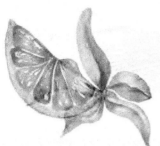

# Weekly Budget

Week

| Item | Budget | Actual |
|------|--------|--------|
|      |        |        |
|      |        |        |
|      |        |        |
|      |        |        |
|      |        |        |
|      |        |        |
|      |        |        |
|      |        |        |
|      |        |        |
|      |        |        |
|      |        |        |
|      |        |        |
|      |        |        |
|      |        |        |
|      |        |        |
|      |        |        |
|      |        |        |
|      |        |        |
|      |        |        |
|      |        |        |
|      |        |        |
|      | TOTAL  |        |

# Weekly Budget

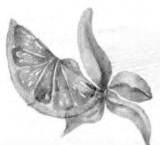

Week

| Item | Budget | Actual |
|---|---|---|
|  |  |  |
|  |  |  |
|  |  |  |
|  |  |  |
|  |  |  |
|  |  |  |
|  |  |  |
|  |  |  |
|  |  |  |
|  |  |  |
|  |  |  |
|  |  |  |
|  |  |  |
|  |  |  |
|  |  |  |
|  |  |  |
|  |  |  |
|  |  |  |
|  |  |  |
|  |  |  |
|  |  |  |
|  |  |  |
| TOTAL |  |  |

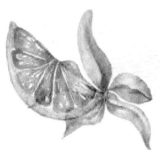

# Weekly Budget

Week

| Item | Budget | Actual |
|---|---|---|
| | | |
| | | |
| | | |
| | | |
| | | |
| | | |
| | | |
| | | |
| | | |
| | | |
| | | |
| | | |
| | | |
| | | |
| | | |
| | | |
| | | |
| | | |
| | | |
| | | |
| | | |
| | | |
| | | |
| | | |
| TOTAL | | |

# Weekly Budget

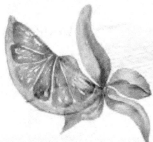

Week

| Item | Budget | Actual |
|---|---|---|
|  |  |  |
|  |  |  |
|  |  |  |
|  |  |  |
|  |  |  |
|  |  |  |
|  |  |  |
|  |  |  |
|  |  |  |
|  |  |  |
|  |  |  |
|  |  |  |
|  |  |  |
|  |  |  |
|  |  |  |
|  |  |  |
|  |  |  |
|  |  |  |
|  |  |  |
|  |  |  |
|  |  |  |
|  |  |  |
| **TOTAL** |  |  |

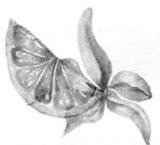

# Weekly Budget

Week

| Item | Budget | Actual |
|---|---|---|
| | | |
| | | |
| | | |
| | | |
| | | |
| | | |
| | | |
| | | |
| | | |
| | | |
| | | |
| | | |
| | | |
| | | |
| | | |
| | | |
| | | |
| | | |
| | | |
| | | |
| | | |
| | | |
| | | |
| | | |
| | | |
| TOTAL | | |

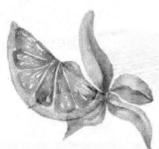

# Weekly Budget

Week

| Item | Budget | | Actual | |
|---|---|---|---|---|
| | | | | |
| | | | | |
| | | | | |
| | | | | |
| | | | | |
| | | | | |
| | | | | |
| | | | | |
| | | | | |
| | | | | |
| | | | | |
| | | | | |
| | | | | |
| | | | | |
| | | | | |
| | | | | |
| | | | | |
| | | | | |
| | | | | |
| | | | | |
| | | | | |
| TOTAL | | | | |

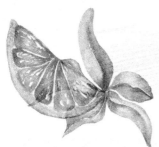

# Weekly Budget

Week

| Item | Budget | Actual |
|---|---|---|
| | | |
| | | |
| | | |
| | | |
| | | |
| | | |
| | | |
| | | |
| | | |
| | | |
| | | |
| | | |
| | | |
| | | |
| | | |
| | | |
| | | |
| | | |
| | | |
| | | |
| | | |
| TOTAL | | |

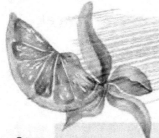

# Pantry Inventory

| Qty | Item | Use by |
|-----|------|--------|
|     |      |        |
|     |      |        |
|     |      |        |
|     |      |        |
|     |      |        |
|     |      |        |
|     |      |        |
|     |      |        |
|     |      |        |
|     |      |        |
|     |      |        |
|     |      |        |
|     |      |        |
|     |      |        |
|     |      |        |
|     |      |        |
|     |      |        |
|     |      |        |
|     |      |        |
|     |      |        |
|     |      |        |
|     |      |        |
|     |      |        |
|     |      |        |
|     |      |        |

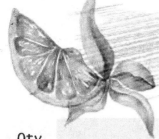

# Pantry Inventory

| Qty | Item | Use by |
|-----|------|--------|
|     |      |        |
|     |      |        |
|     |      |        |
|     |      |        |
|     |      |        |
|     |      |        |
|     |      |        |
|     |      |        |
|     |      |        |
|     |      |        |
|     |      |        |
|     |      |        |
|     |      |        |
|     |      |        |
|     |      |        |
|     |      |        |
|     |      |        |
|     |      |        |
|     |      |        |
|     |      |        |
|     |      |        |
|     |      |        |
|     |      |        |
|     |      |        |
|     |      |        |
|     |      |        |
|     |      |        |

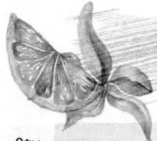

# Fridge Inventory

| Qty | Item | Use by |
|-----|------|--------|
|     |      |        |
|     |      |        |
|     |      |        |
|     |      |        |
|     |      |        |
|     |      |        |
|     |      |        |
|     |      |        |
|     |      |        |
|     |      |        |
|     |      |        |
|     |      |        |
|     |      |        |
|     |      |        |
|     |      |        |
|     |      |        |
|     |      |        |
|     |      |        |
|     |      |        |
|     |      |        |
|     |      |        |
|     |      |        |
|     |      |        |
|     |      |        |

# Fridge Inventory

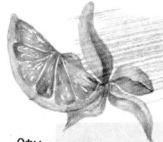

| Qty | Item | Use by |
|-----|------|--------|
|     |      |        |
|     |      |        |
|     |      |        |
|     |      |        |
|     |      |        |
|     |      |        |
|     |      |        |
|     |      |        |
|     |      |        |
|     |      |        |
|     |      |        |
|     |      |        |
|     |      |        |
|     |      |        |
|     |      |        |
|     |      |        |
|     |      |        |
|     |      |        |
|     |      |        |
|     |      |        |
|     |      |        |
|     |      |        |
|     |      |        |
|     |      |        |
|     |      |        |
|     |      |        |

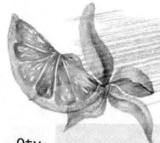

# Freezer Inventory

| Qty | Item | Use by |
|-----|------|--------|
|     |      |        |
|     |      |        |
|     |      |        |
|     |      |        |
|     |      |        |
|     |      |        |
|     |      |        |
|     |      |        |
|     |      |        |
|     |      |        |
|     |      |        |
|     |      |        |
|     |      |        |
|     |      |        |
|     |      |        |
|     |      |        |
|     |      |        |
|     |      |        |
|     |      |        |
|     |      |        |
|     |      |        |
|     |      |        |
|     |      |        |
|     |      |        |
|     |      |        |
|     |      |        |
|     |      |        |
|     |      |        |
|     |      |        |
|     |      |        |

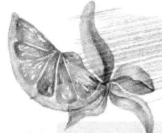

# Freezer Inventory

| Qty | Item | Use by |
|-----|------|--------|
|     |      |        |
|     |      |        |
|     |      |        |
|     |      |        |
|     |      |        |
|     |      |        |
|     |      |        |
|     |      |        |
|     |      |        |
|     |      |        |
|     |      |        |
|     |      |        |
|     |      |        |
|     |      |        |
|     |      |        |
|     |      |        |
|     |      |        |
|     |      |        |
|     |      |        |
|     |      |        |
|     |      |        |
|     |      |        |
|     |      |        |
|     |      |        |
|     |      |        |
|     |      |        |
|     |      |        |
|     |      |        |

# Breakfast Ideas

**WEEK 1**

**WEEK 2**

# Breakfast Ideas

**WEEK 3**

**WEEK 4**

# Breakfast Ideas

WEEK 5

WEEK 6

# Breakfast Ideas

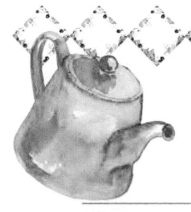

**WEEK 7**

**WEEK 8**

# Breakfast Ideas

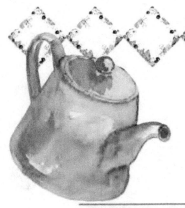

**WEEK 9**

**WEEK 10**

# Breakfast Ideas

**WEEK 11**

**WEEK 12**

# Breakfast Ideas

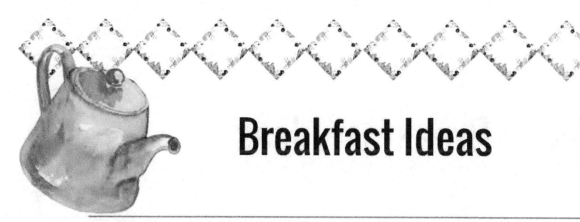

**WEEK**

**WEEK**

# Breakfast Ideas

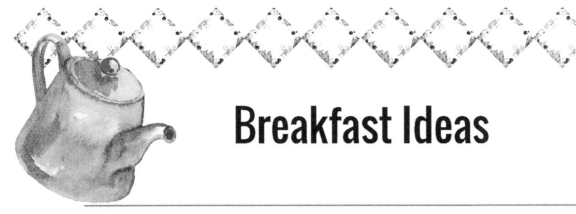

**WEEK**

**WEEK**

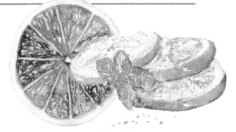

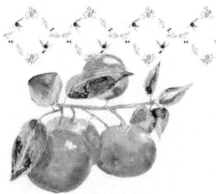
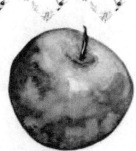

# Lunch Ideas

**WEEK 1**

**WEEK 2**

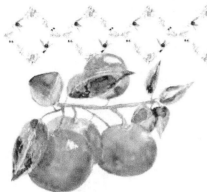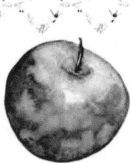

# Lunch Ideas

**WEEK 3**

**WEEK 4**

# Lunch Ideas

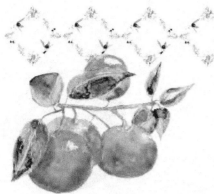
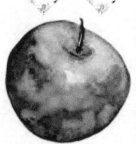

**WEEK 5**

**WEEK 6**

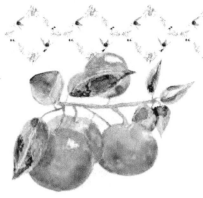
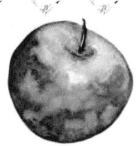

# Lunch Ideas

**WEEK 7**

**WEEK 8**

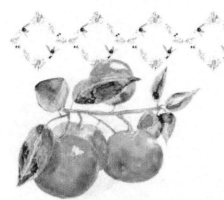
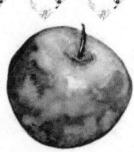

# Lunch Ideas

**WEEK 9**

**WEEK 10**

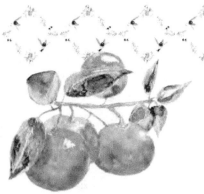
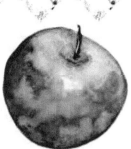

# Lunch Ideas

**WEEK 11**

**WEEK 12**

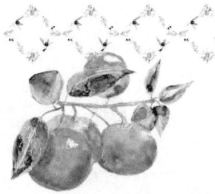
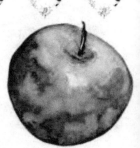

# Lunch Ideas

**WEEK**

**WEEK**

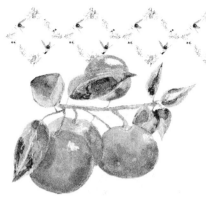
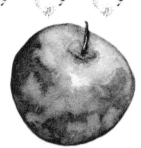

# Lunch Ideas

**WEEK**

**WEEK**

# Dinner Ideas

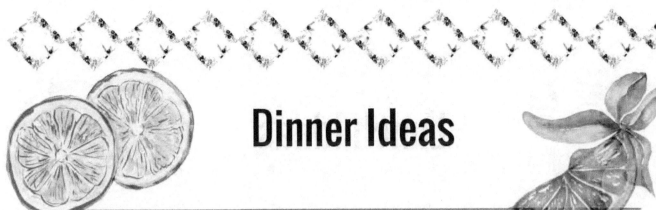

**WEEK 1**

**WEEK 2**

# Dinner Ideas

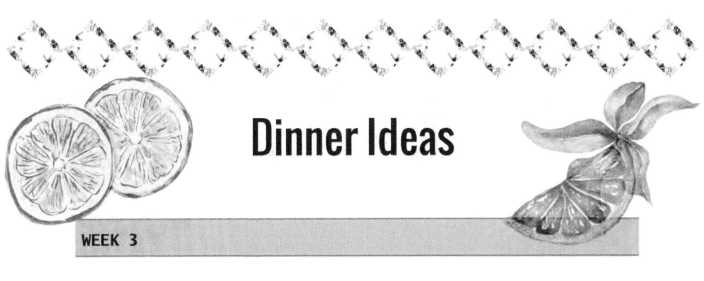

**WEEK 3**

**WEEK 4**

# Dinner Ideas

**WEEK 5**

**WEEK 6**

# Dinner Ideas

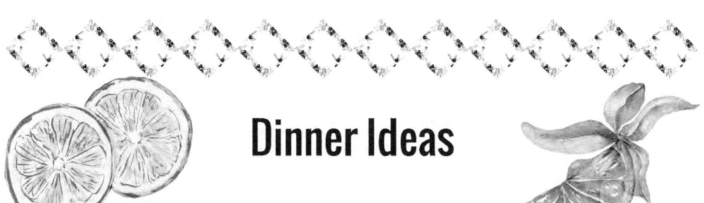

**WEEK 7**

**WEEK 8**

# Dinner Ideas

**WEEK 9**

**WEEK 10**

# Dinner Ideas

**WEEK 11**

**WEEK 12**

# Dinner Ideas

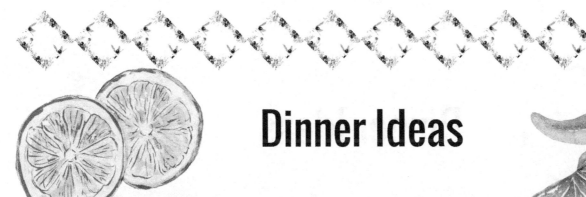

**WEEK**

**WEEK**

# Dinner Ideas

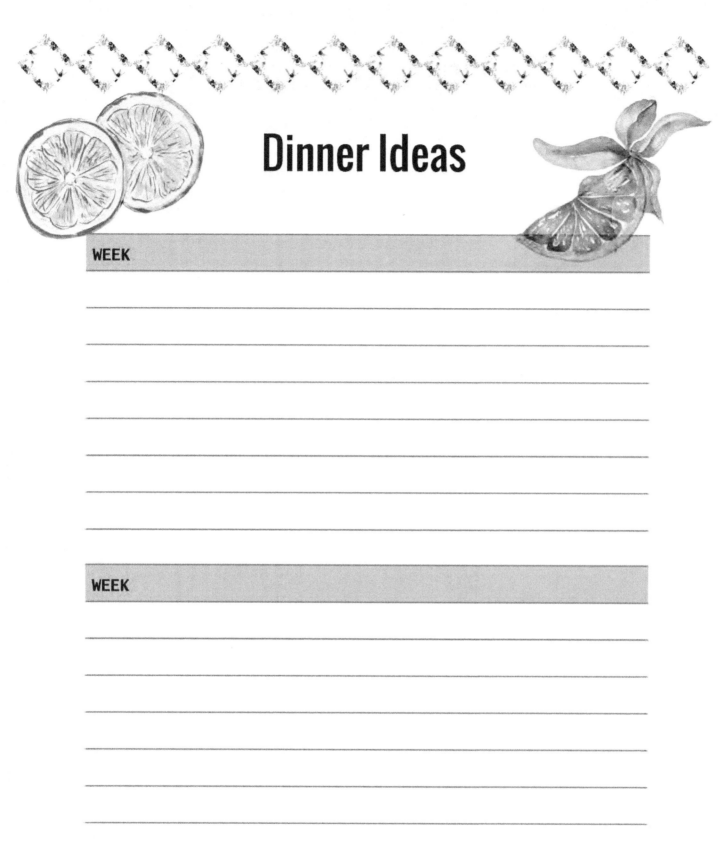

**WEEK**

**WEEK**

# Dealing with Leftovers

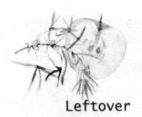 

| Leftover | Description |
|----------|-------------|
|          |             |
|          |             |
|          |             |
|          |             |
|          |             |
|          |             |
|          |             |

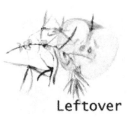
# Dealing with Leftovers

Leftover | Description

# Ideas for Snacks

| Snack | Ingredients |
|-------|-------------|
|       |             |
|       |             |
|       |             |
|       |             |
|       |             |
|       |             |
|       |             |

# Ideas for Snacks

| Snack | Ingredients |
|-------|-------------|
|       |             |
|       |             |
|       |             |
|       |             |
|       |             |
|       |             |

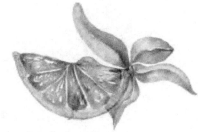

# Healthy Fast Food

| Outlet | Speciality | Contact No. |
|---|---|---|
| | | |

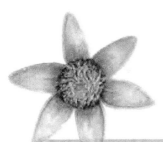
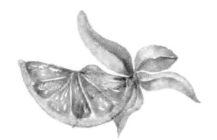

# Healthy Fast Food

| Outlet | Speciality | Contact No. |
| --- | --- | --- |

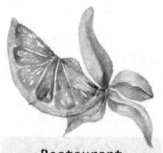
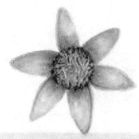

# Dining Out

| Restaurant | Speciality | Contact No. | Family Rating |
|---|---|---|---|
| | | | ☆ ☆ ☆ ☆ ☆ |
| | | | ☆ ☆ ☆ ☆ ☆ |
| | | | ☆ ☆ ☆ ☆ ☆ |
| | | | ☆ ☆ ☆ ☆ ☆ |
| | | | ☆ ☆ ☆ ☆ ☆ |
| | | | ☆ ☆ ☆ ☆ ☆ |
| | | | ☆ ☆ ☆ ☆ ☆ |
| | | | ☆ ☆ ☆ ☆ ☆ |
| | | | ☆ ☆ ☆ ☆ ☆ |
| | | | ☆ ☆ ☆ ☆ ☆ |
| | | | ☆ ☆ ☆ ☆ ☆ |
| | | | ☆ ☆ ☆ ☆ ☆ |
| | | | ☆ ☆ ☆ ☆ ☆ |
| | | | ☆ ☆ ☆ ☆ ☆ |
| | | | ☆ ☆ ☆ ☆ ☆ |
| | | | ☆ ☆ ☆ ☆ ☆ |
| | | | ☆ ☆ ☆ ☆ ☆ |
| | | | ☆ ☆ ☆ ☆ ☆ |
| | | | ☆ ☆ ☆ ☆ ☆ |

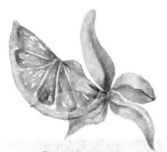

# Dining Out

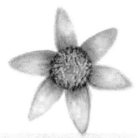

| Restaurant | Speciality | Contact No. | Family Rating |
|---|---|---|---|
| | | | ☆ ☆ ☆ ☆ ☆ |
| | | | ☆ ☆ ☆ ☆ ☆ |
| | | | ☆ ☆ ☆ ☆ ☆ |
| | | | ☆ ☆ ☆ ☆ ☆ |
| | | | ☆ ☆ ☆ ☆ ☆ |
| | | | ☆ ☆ ☆ ☆ ☆ |
| | | | ☆ ☆ ☆ ☆ ☆ |
| | | | ☆ ☆ ☆ ☆ ☆ |
| | | | ☆ ☆ ☆ ☆ ☆ |
| | | | ☆ ☆ ☆ ☆ ☆ |
| | | | ☆ ☆ ☆ ☆ ☆ |
| | | | ☆ ☆ ☆ ☆ ☆ |
| | | | ☆ ☆ ☆ ☆ ☆ |
| | | | ☆ ☆ ☆ ☆ ☆ |
| | | | ☆ ☆ ☆ ☆ ☆ |
| | | | ☆ ☆ ☆ ☆ ☆ |
| | | | ☆ ☆ ☆ ☆ ☆ |
| | | | ☆ ☆ ☆ ☆ ☆ |
| | | | ☆ ☆ ☆ ☆ ☆ |

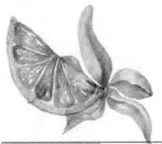
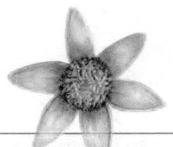

# Entertaining

| Date | | Occasion | |
|---|---|---|---|

## Guest List

| Name | Likes | Dislikes | Allergies |
|---|---|---|---|
|  |  |  |  |
|  |  |  |  |
|  |  |  |  |
|  |  |  |  |
|  |  |  |  |
|  |  |  |  |
|  |  |  |  |
|  |  |  |  |
|  |  |  |  |
|  |  |  |  |

**Menu**

| To Do | To Buy |
|---|---|
|  |  |
|  |  |
|  |  |
|  |  |
|  |  |
|  |  |

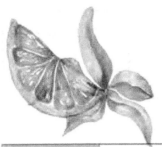
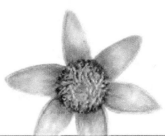

# Entertaining

| Date | | Occasion | |

## Guest List

| Name | Likes | Dislikes | Allergies |
|------|-------|----------|-----------|
|      |       |          |           |
|      |       |          |           |
|      |       |          |           |
|      |       |          |           |
|      |       |          |           |
|      |       |          |           |
|      |       |          |           |
|      |       |          |           |
|      |       |          |           |
|      |       |          |           |

## Menu

| To Do | To Buy |
|-------|--------|
|       |        |
|       |        |
|       |        |
|       |        |
|       |        |
|       |        |

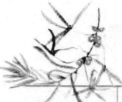

# Holiday Meal Planner

Holiday

**Menu**
- Starter
- Main
- Dessert
- Snacks
- Drinks

| Décor | People at the Table |
|---|---|
|  |  |
|  |  |
|  |  |
|  |  |

| Preparation Checklist | | To Do | To Buy |
|---|---|---|---|
| Date | Details | | |
|  |  | ○ | ○ |
|  |  | ○ | ○ |
|  |  | ○ | ○ |
|  |  | ○ | ○ |
|  |  | ○ | ○ |
|  |  | ○ | ○ |
|  |  | ○ | ○ |
|  |  | ○ | ○ |
|  |  | ○ | ○ |
|  |  | ○ | ○ |
|  |  | ○ | ○ |
|  |  | ○ | ○ |

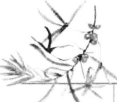

# Holiday Meal Planner

Holiday

| Menu | |
|---|---|
| | Starter |
| | Main |
| | Dessert |
| | Snacks |
| | Drinks |

| Décor | People at the Table |
|---|---|
| | |
| | |
| | |
| | |

| Preparation Checklist | | To Do | To Buy |
|---|---|---|---|
| Date | Details | | |
| | | ○ | ○ |
| | | ○ | ○ |
| | | ○ | ○ |
| | | ○ | ○ |
| | | ○ | ○ |
| | | ○ | ○ |
| | | ○ | ○ |
| | | ○ | ○ |
| | | ○ | ○ |
| | | ○ | ○ |
| | | ○ | ○ |
| | | ○ | ○ |

# Family Favorite Meals

## Spring

_____
_____
_____
_____
_____
_____
_____

## Summer

_____
_____
_____
_____
_____
_____
_____

## Autumn

_____
_____
_____
_____
_____
_____
_____

## Winter

_____
_____
_____
_____
_____
_____
_____

# Family Favorite Meals

Spring

Summer

Autumn

Winter

# Likes and Dislikes

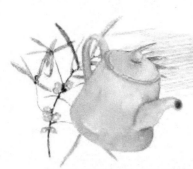
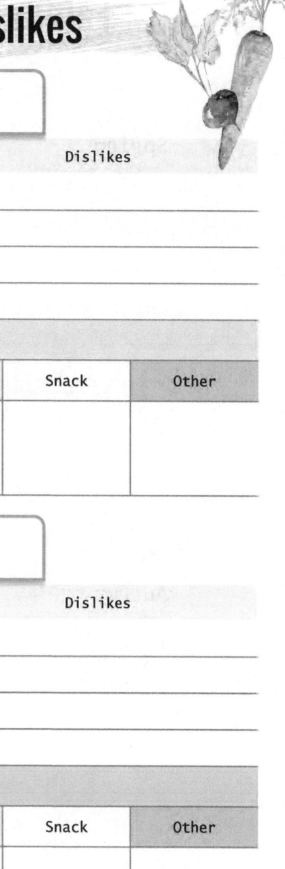

**Name**

| Likes | Dislikes |
|---|---|
|  |  |
|  |  |
|  |  |

### Favorite

| Breakfast | Lunch | Dinner | Snack | Other |
|---|---|---|---|---|
|  |  |  |  |  |

**Name**

| Likes | Dislikes |
|---|---|
|  |  |
|  |  |
|  |  |

### Favorite

| Breakfast | Lunch | Dinner | Snack | Other |
|---|---|---|---|---|
|  |  |  |  |  |

# Likes and Dislikes

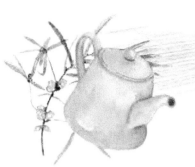
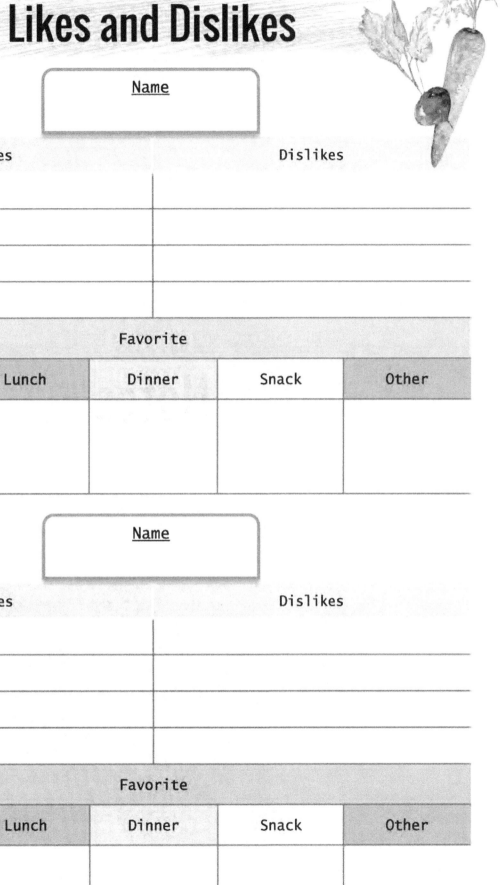

**Name**

| Likes | Dislikes |
|---|---|
| | |
| | |
| | |

### Favorite

| Breakfast | Lunch | Dinner | Snack | Other |
|---|---|---|---|---|
| | | | | |

**Name**

| Likes | Dislikes |
|---|---|
| | |
| | |
| | |

### Favorite

| Breakfast | Lunch | Dinner | Snack | Other |
|---|---|---|---|---|
| | | | | |

# Notes

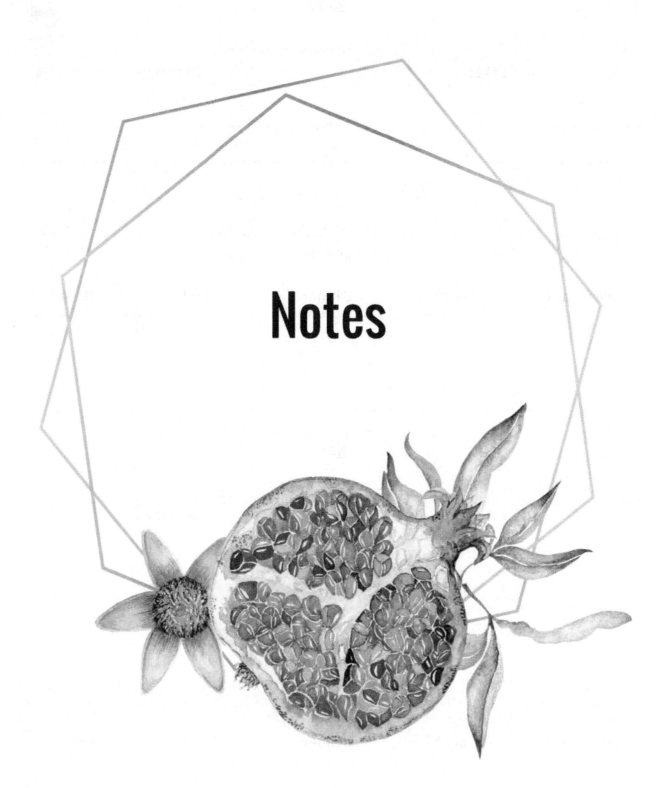

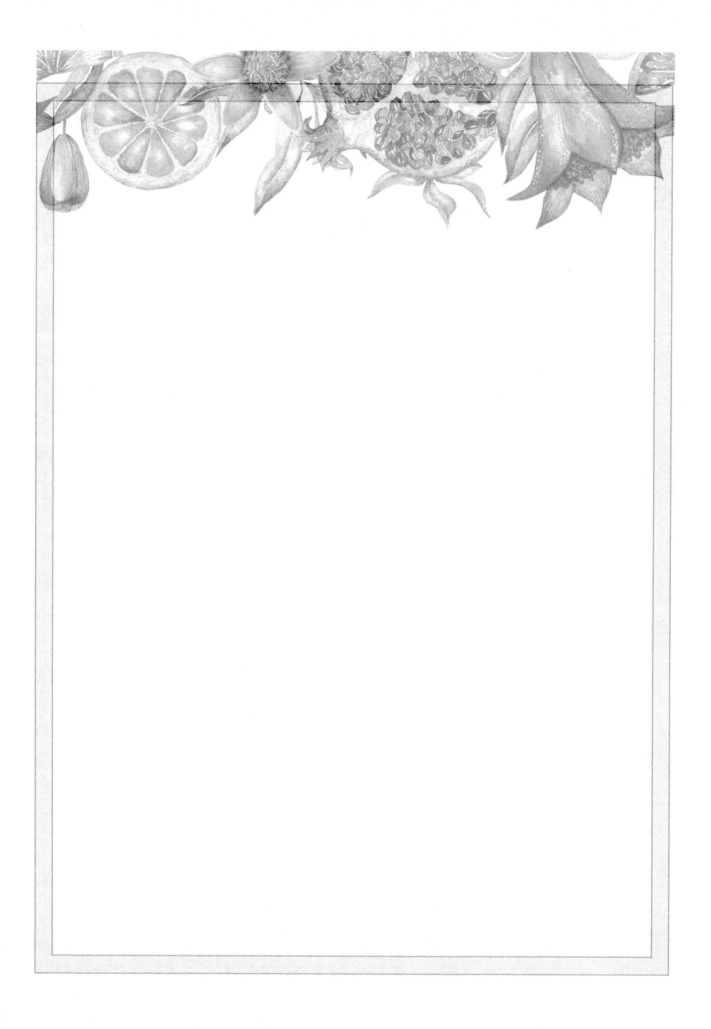

For more health-related journals and planners please visit:
https://healthylivingideas.ca/healthy-living-journal-store/
or stop by at my author page as I add more journals and planners to my collection:
https://www.amazon.com/author/healthylivingjournals

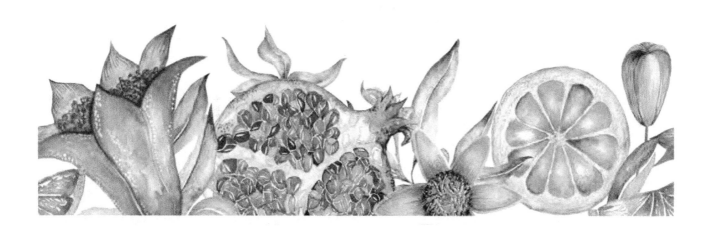

Made in the USA
Monee, IL
25 February 2025